Fighting *for* Joy

Fighting *for* Joy

My Breast Cancer Journey

by
Jennifer Hooper

Hardcover ISBN: 978-0-57894-672-6
Digital ISBN: 978-0-57894-673-3

Fighting For Joy:
My Breast Cancer Journey

Connect on Instagram
@jendhooper

Table of Contents

Dedication

Introduction

Dedication:

This book is dedicated to all those currently fighting cancer, and to all those who were my support system during my journey.

"I know I have access to all that He is and all that He provides because He lives in me. And I know that if He asks me to do something unexpected, He's already gone before me."

~Christine Caine (Unexpected)

Introduction:

Hi friends! I'm Jennifer. At the time of writing this, I'm 35 years old, a wife, married 14 years to my best friend, Tim, and a mother of 4 sweet kiddos (2 boys, 2 girls, ages 6-11). My sweet friend, Courtney, and I host a podcast called *Enough*. Tim and I have a ministry called *The Journey Home* where we have the privilege of loving on couples and leaders who are on the brink of burnout in an off-the-grid, judgment-free place. Most importantly, I'm completely in love with Jesus and desire nothing more than to love on women and show them how amazing they are, how loved and accepted they are, and how completely confident they can rest in this because of Jesus.

First of all, if you are currently fighting cancer, my heart aches for you. I wish I could give you a HUGE hug, look you in the eye and tell you that I know it's scary. I know you're afraid, and that's ok. I also want to tell you that God knew this was part of your story and He has been preparing you for this. He's got you and HE WILL NOT LET GO!! Look up my friend and keep your eyes on Jesus!

If you're reading this book and have a loved one that is currently suffering from cancer, I'm glad you're here. I pray this book will help you to understand a little better what they're going through and will encourage you as well, because as a caretaker, there's a load you're carrying that's often just as heavy.

The purpose of this book is to inspire hope that it *is* possible to keep your eyes on Jesus in the storm. Everything in this book is not to tell you what to do if you're currently in your battle with cancer, it's simply my story. Your story will be completely different because there are no two people alike. But, there is one thing that IS the same ... JESUS IS WITH YOU!

I get pretty raw and personal in this book with everything that I have felt throughout this process in hopes that you feel that you're not alone with your fears.

I share my story not because of its uniqueness or profoundness, but because I felt God ask me to share my story. Your story will look entirely different and will be just as unique and profound. Many people choose to keep silent about their breast cancer because of the intimate nature of this kind of cancer and that is completely understandable. My desire is you will see God woven throughout every word so that He gets the glory and so that any strength you feel that I have, you can have too, by God's grace.

~Jen

Part 1

My Story

Chapter 1

"It's Cancer"

In December of 2019, I discovered a bump on my chest located on the right side that protruded quite a bit and was pretty visible. I chalked it up to something muscular because of the location of the bump and the fact that I'd been struggling with some pretty bad knots directly behind it on my back.

But first, I need to give you a little back story of what God was doing in my heart. I've always been a very shy person - very introverted ... like SCARED to speak. I would stumble over my words and always felt like what I had to say wasn't important. Well, after years of craving to be used by God, I felt Him telling me that He wanted to use my voice. And ... I laughed. I know, I know ... not a good idea. But God in His mercy, gently told me (not audibly, but a whisper in my heart), "How much more glory can I get when you can't get the glory", because you see, I don't have what it takes, BUT Jesus IN me does!

"I can do all things through Christ who strengthens me." So, I told God, if He could use my voice, it's all His.

A day or two later, I saw a post on Instagram from a lady that I had messaged occasionally and was beginning to really respect for her love for Jesus. I knew in my heart that we would do something together one day, I just didn't know what. Well, this post was about her launching a t-shirt she had designed that said, "Enough", and she shared how this word meant a lot to her because in her curly hair journey it was teaching her that she was enough because Jesus made her enough. That was it! I messaged her immediately and shared what God was doing in my heart and that I knew it sounded crazy, but I felt that God wanted us to do something together that had to do with our identity in Christ. Because of God's timing she messaged back and said, "Let's do a podcast". Immediately I knew this was it! That is just like God to ask you to do something, but still allow you to live in your strengths. He didn't ask me to go on the road and speak on a stage that would COMPLETELY terrify me. He asked me to be behind a microphone in the comfort of my own home with the beautiful power of editing. Lol!

A friend of my husband had a podcast and was so sweet in her willingness to teach me how to podcast.

So, we flew from Central Virginia to California just to learn how to podcast ... crazy, I know! But, I knew God was in it. However, I ended up with a nasty ear infection right before our flight and the antibiotic was not doing its job even after five days. I knew with the pressure of the airplane, this was not going to be a fun flight. BUT GOD ... the second I stepped on the airplane, my earache was GONE!!

Two months later, in April of 2020, and I have another earache. This time I was trying to go the natural route to get rid of it, but it spread to the other ear and I began to feel a twinge in the first ear. One morning preparing to record a podcast with my friend, she highly encouraged me to get it checked out. I decided to also get this bump checked out for peace of mind. I was convinced that it was nothing. Maybe a cyst or I was going to need needle therapy (thinking it was the knots in my back) ... I HATE needles! My doctor sent me to UVA (University of Virginia) Cancer Center for an ultrasound, which seemed to take FOREVER. Finally, the doctor finished and said they also wanted a mammogram. At this point, red flags are starting to go up. After what seemed like more pictures than necessary, another doctor came in and told me they wanted to do another ultrasound and that when it was done they promised we would talk. Tears started to flow during this ultrasound knowing that this wasn't looking good. He said that he didn't like what he saw and that there was another spot that looked concerning. They wanted to do a biopsy and I asked if my husband could come in with me and hear what the doctor had to say because I was afraid I wouldn't be able to retain the information. Because of the COVID19 pandemic, and our state at the time being at a level of extreme caution, it was a miracle they actually let Tim in. They scheduled my biopsy for the next day. I ended up having a biopsy on three different locations on my right side.

I had no idea what a biopsy even was and I was terrified. In case you haven't gotten the hint yet (LOL), I get super squeamish regarding needles or when you start talking about ANY kind of procedure. In fact, I passed out the first time they drew blood when I was pregnant with my oldest child. Even the retaining guard they use (which reminds me of a school desk) didn't hold me. Yep, I slid right under the guard, out of that seat and onto the floor. Ok ... so you get the picture? Now, back to the biopsy. I almost had a panic attack walking into the doctor's office. As I'm writing this, I'm starting to shake again just remembering those feelings. BUT GOD, showed up in that room in a very real way. Not only did I see Jesus in the eyes of one of the doctors and nurse, but they also turned on worship music for me. One of the songs that came on was "In Christ Alone". As they started the procedure, I had this amazing peace wash over me. I went from fidgety and feeling like I was going to pass out to completely still. I felt as if I were laying right at Jesus' feet. Anytime I would start to think about what the doctors were doing, I would feel Jesus whispering, "No, I'm right here. Take my hand. I've got you!" And peace would sweep over me again. It was a moment I will never forget.

I love how Becky Thompson in her book, *Peace*, explains how miracles happen. The feeding of the five thousand didn't have an endless supply of bread and fish. There was an end to it, along with many other miracles in the Bible. I believe this shows us that we will always have a continual need for Christ. He didn't give me endless peace. He gave me peace in the moment I needed it most. All that to say, when I got home it was a healing process that I wasn't expecting. The nurse told me before I left that I was not allowed to lift over a half-gallon of milk and that I COULD NOT STIR or any other repetitive motion. Y'ALL!!!! Baking is my thing! I absolutely LOVE getting in the kitchen and baking cookies and cakes. Stirring is kind of a prerequisite for baking. But not only that, I couldn't seem to shake the feeling in my chest and a squeamish sort of pain that lasted for several days. It was a constant reminder of what I had just been through and the fear of the unknown. What is it? Is it cancer? Is it benign? My family and friends were praying for the latter, but I was conflicted as to how to pray. I just wanted God's will. Whatever He chose. Personally I didn't want to go through cancer, surgery, or whatever else might be on the horizon. But, I had a feeling in my gut that wouldn't go away.

That Sunday, we watched a sermon about finding joy in trials by Andy Stanley. A heaviness swept over me like I'd never felt before and by the end of the message, I couldn't stop crying. Tim and my mom came around me and were trying to console me and tell me that everything was going to be ok. But I knew! I had cancer! I felt so strongly that, between our ministry at *The Journey Home* and our *Enough* podcast and my intense desire to encourage women in our identity in Christ, God wanted me to walk through this so I could feel it for others and I was to take note of my feelings and thoughts through the process. I felt the weight of what I was about to go through along with an intense gratitude that God was entrusting this journey to me. He was giving me a voice. Without realizing it, I had "asked" for this. Not the answer I would have preferred obviously (and on the onset, it's difficult to see any trial as an answer to prayer); but my intense desire has been to serve God and bring Him glory ... whatever the cost. Tim and my mom were praying that I was wrong. But the next day, May 18th, 2020 the call came. It was breast cancer. The praise was that my lymph nodes were clear of cancer, but a second spot (although it didn't appear to be cancerous) still didn't look right. My body was shaking uncontrollably like it knew what I was about to experience, but my mind was strong. I felt a wave of gratitude sweep over me and I genuinely felt that God gave me a gift. I felt honored (and still feel so humbled and grateful) that God entrusted me with this journey. God has given me a supernatural amount of strength and peace. I can only give praise to Jesus for my mindset during this time. I was ready to drop to my knees and give Him praise while also dreading what I was about to walk through.

About a week later I took off my final Band-aid from the biopsy and I started shaking uncontrollably envisioning what it would look like after my surgery. I sat in front of my window overlooking the Blue Ridge Mountains. I opened the window, breathed in deeply smelling the pines and listened to the birds. It sounded like they were worshipping Jesus and I realized I just needed to worship Jesus, too. Honestly, it's always worship that gives me the hope and peace I need.

Chapter 2

What's Next?

To preface this chapter I would like to say, once again, that everything in this book is my experience and recalling my story. This is not a recommendation for what you should do. You are unique and your story will be unique.

After my next visit to UVA, I found out that I would definitely undergo surgery, and they strongly advised hormone therapy after. Next step was to get an MRI to find out if I would be having a mastectomy (full removal of the breast), or lumpectomy (removing just the lump). I don't have the words to describe the feelings standing on that mat in front of a massive door that led into the room to get my MRI. Seeing all the hazard signs, waiting for the door to release before it opened, and seeing other people waiting at other doors was a very somber experience.

One of the hardest things about this part of my story was all the decisions to make. I was afraid if I made the wrong decision it would mean more doctor visits and additional surgeries. It's amazing to me, though, that God will tell you every tiny detail you need to know if you listen. God knows your body better than any doctor, and even better than you do. Listen, and He will guide you through anything you need to know. I found out that I had HER2- which was huge because this meant I may not need chemo. Although my doctor told me I would most likely need a mastectomy, I could also choose to do another biopsy to further discover if just a lumpectomy with radiation would suffice. I chose to go with the mastectomy because of the second spot, and honestly, I didn't want to go through another biopsy only to come to the realization that I still needed a mastectomy.

The idea of a mastectomy terrified me! The fact of having to remove an entire part of me was devastating. Not only because of body image, but also because I feared how I would feel as a wife. Let me also say that it is a strain on any marriage when you are going through surgery recovery, pregnancy, or any other life circumstance that prevents intimacy. One thing that helped Tim and I the most through four pregnancies and now surgery was talking to each other. Be honest and keep that line of communication open.

Ok, back to the story. I now had more decisions to make. Would I go with implants or tissue reconstruction (where they remove tissue from one part of your body, in my case my stomach, and reconstruct your breast)? Then God brought my hair and skin journey to mind. A year prior to my diagnosis, I started to learn about how to care for my naturally curly hair. I began learning more about the ingredients of products, stopped straightening my hair (learning that heat could damage it), and using tips and tricks to style my hair. After a year of doing this, my hair was the healthiest it had ever been. I realized through this journey and with a lot of research that my hair didn't like silicones and also in playing around with different skin products, I found out that my skin didn't like silicones either. I believe that because of my hair journey and learning about my skin not agreeing with silicones, God was telling me what my body needed. So, I decided against implants, and chose tissue reconstruction. Unfortunately, this was also the hardest route for me, because it completely grossed me out, and I knew it meant a longer and harder recovery, not to mention longer, more-extensive surgery. But, in hind sight, I'm thankful I chose tissue reconstruction because more than likely I won't need additional surgeries ten to fifteen years down the road to maintain implants.

During the decision-making process - MRI, CT scan, and many doctor consultations - so much was happening in my mind and heart. I remember after my first consultation with the plastic surgeon, everything hit me HARD. However, the messages of many women being inspired by my story continued to give me purpose and reminded me that I was walking this journey to feel the full weight of what so many women walk through. It was important to me to keep my spiritual eyes open and fixed on Jesus.

I know there are many natural options out there and many people believe you should go a natural route. In fact, this route was very tempting for me. A strict, clean diet to replace needles and surgery? Yes please! However, I believe God gives doctors wisdom and can use all of it - medicine and nutrition. For my journey, I was fully convinced and felt peace that I needed to feel what a majority of women have felt - the pain and loss of going through with surgery. Especially, considering the higher-risk and fast-growth nature of my cancer, and that I was persuaded this was God's plan for my story. I know so many people are well-meaning and really care, but truthfully, some messages and "advice" can hurt and even feel judgmental that you didn't choose a "better" route. I want to reach through these pages and assure you there is NO PERFECT route when you're dealing with the devastating news of cancer; BUT, there is a PERFECT Healer who can and does use it all! So listen to your doctors, eat cleaner, do what you can, and most importantly trust God! Again, this is my story and what I knew God wanted me to experience. Every single woman that has had breast cancer is going to have a different story and I am not recommending anything, just sharing my journey and what God was doing inside of me.

Isaiah 43:1-2

"But now thus says the LORD, he who created you,
O Jacob, he who formed you, O Israel:

'Fear not, for I have redeemed you; I have called
you by name, you are mine.

When you pass through the waters, I will be
with you; and through the rivers, they shall not
overwhelm you;

when you walk through fire you shall not be burned,
and the flame shall not consume you.'"

Chapter 3

Fear Not

When we got the call that I had cancer, our Pastor called to pray with us. He ended the conversation with a verse that hadn't been prevalent in my mind for a while, but has become the verse that I've clung to throughout this journey.

Isaiah 43:1-2 - "But now thus saith the LORD that created you, O Jacob, and he that formed you, O Israel, Fear not: for I have redeemed you, I have called you by name; you are mine. When you pass through the waters, I will be with you; and through the rivers, they will not overflow you: when you walk through the fire, you will not be burned; neither will the flame kindle upon you."

A few days later, we were introduced to a new crowd-funded series called *The Chosen*. It's probably the most well-done series based on the life of Christ I've ever seen. Mostly because it makes me think a little differently about the stories we read in the Bible. It makes them come to life and helps me realize that they were regular people like you and me who had their own struggles and insecurities. The first episode was about Mary Magdalene - a complete tear jerker - because it gives a little more insight into how things might've been during that time in history. At the very end of the episode Jesus heals her, and what verse did they use throughout this episode? You guessed it! Isa. 43:1 "I have called you by name ... You are mine"!

On Tim's and my very next drive to UVA, we turn on our worship music and the song, *Be Not Afraid,* came on over the car's speaker! The song is taken from Isaiah 43:1-2! I don't know about you, but God has a way of confirming in three's for me!!! Not saying it has to be three - it might be more or less - but one thing I CAN guarantee is God promises He will never leave you or forsake you! He says, "You are MINE"! He promises that no matter what you walk through, He will be with you! This verse has become a battle cry for me and my family.

Fear is inevitable in a journey like this and let me be clear - feeling fear is NOT wrong. Why else would He say over and over in Scripture "Fear not" if we didn't feel fear? But, what are you choosing to do with fear? Let it control you, or courageously continue to move forward in boldness knowing that God has your back? I felt fear every day of this journey. But, I didn't and I won't allow it to hold me down.

I can't tell you why sometimes it feels like we're all alone, even when we know God is with us. Sometimes we feel His presence so close, but other times it feels as though He's far away. It might be because we took our eyes off of Him and put them on the waves around us like Peter; but, there are also times that I've been straining to keep my eyes focused on Him and I still feel alone. Why does this happen? I don't know the answer to that question; however, from personal experience, He has always showed up. Not when I thought He should, but in His timing. Actually, it's always the perfect timing. I've found that the harder I fight to keep my eyes on Him - and by that I mean playing worship music and singing in my heart meaning every word, reading my Bible, repeating scripture over and over, or taking a walk, looking up and breathing in His creation - the more I've felt rewarded for fighting to stand firm and not take my eyes off of Him.

I think about how David "encouraged himself in the Lord". Sometimes there might not be someone around you to speak truth over you, but that's when you have to allow God's voice to drown out all the fear and lies. True courage is continuing to move forward, continuing to get out of bed in the morning when you're paralyzed in fear. Ask God to give you the courage that you know you don't have. True courage is continuing to walk boldly *through* the fear.

Chapter 4

Speak Up

July 9th, 2020. Surgery day was here. I'd prepared my body emotionally and physically to the best of my ability. Up to this point, Tim hadn't been allowed to come in with me for any more appointments; but, two weeks before my surgery, our state went from phase-2 to phase-3 of re-opening from the Coronavirus which allowed Tim to come in with me as they prepped me for surgery. Being able to hold his hand that morning and pray together was very special for me, and for him. They did a nerve block instead of doing so many pain killers, which I had great success with. Right after they hooked everything up and confirmed my personal info and type of surgeries they would be performing over the next eight hours, they had Tim head down to the main lobby where he would wait. They got the nerve block going and I began to feel myself going out of consciousness. I woke up slightly as they wheeled me into what I believe was the operating room. I couldn't really see anything so it's just an educated guess. But, all that was going through my mind was, "Say Jesus' name ... say it louder ... say it again!" So I just kept repeating, "I love my Jesus. Jesus is so good to me." I kept hearing in my heart, "Say it again. Say it louder." Until I heard what was probably one of the nurses say, "I love Jesus, too." I started to cry; then I fell asleep. When I woke up, it felt like only five minutes had passed and all I could think of was, "No, I don't want to wake up yet. Surely they're not done yet. I don't want to see this." LOL ... but sure enough, it was done and it had actually been the full eight hours.

What happened to me during that time and what I felt in those moments, I will never forget. As I heard, "say Jesus' name" over and over, and "say it louder", for once in my life I didn't care how I sounded, what I looked like or who was listening! I just wanted to say Jesus' name. And I felt God asking me to speak up. I want to spend the rest of my life saying Jesus' name as loud and as much as I can.

The healing process was very long and at times I felt like I was going crazy. Because honestly, what mama wants to spend four weeks barely able to move; another four weeks before feeling like I could move around somewhat normally; and still, another four weeks before I could get back into my normal routine.

The drains were definitely the hardest part of the healing process. I had three, and boy was it a struggle to figure out what to do with those things any time I got out of bed. Plus, they COMPLETELY grossed me out and I could barely even look at them without seizing up in fear. Then came the cleaning of the drains. UGH!! I spent many a time saying my verse, Isaiah 43:1-2, crying out with an ugly cry and trying - emphasis on *trying* - to sing, *Be Not Afraid* (taken from Isa. 43:1-2). It wasn't pretty, but it helped. It kept me from passing out, and it shifted my focus from the disgusting feeling to my Jesus who was walking with me. He promised me that when I walked through the waters, He would be with me: and through the rivers, they would not sweep over me: when I walk through the fire, I would not be burned. I decided to take Him at His word and trust that He was right there with me. I knew He was, because He promised.

I would like to talk about triggers for a minute. I underestimated how much impact the actual surgery had on my mind. I was watching my favorite Hallmark series, *Signed, Sealed, Delivered,* one day while chilling in bed. It was a scene of someone getting wheeled into the operating room for surgery and I completely lost it. I started sobbing uncontrollably. You never know when a trigger will hit you and this applies not only to surgery, but also to cancer in general and multiple other things. I want you to know that in any moment a trigger hits you, you are held! It feels as though everything is crashing in around you, but the truth is, you are being held by God Almighty! Deuteronomy 23:27 "The eternal God is your dwelling place, and underneath are the everlasting arms"! I will also say that it does *not* help to stuff your feelings! The best way to handle a trigger is by allowing yourself to feel *everything*! Yes, sometimes you just have to buckle up and wait until a private moment when you can allow yourself to feel the full weight of what is happening. But let me give you permission that you don't have to be strong and hold it all together! Something I had to continuously remind myself of when people would tell me what an inspiration I was, or when people would comment on my smile, was that I can still show my weaknesses. When I wasn't feeling ok, I was honest with that fact; but, I'd also share what I knew was truth. That God is good ... all the time! When you decide to stuff your feelings, they're going to come back up eventually. But, it's so much harder the longer you continue to stuff them. Be open. Find someone who will allow you to be raw and real. Someone who will listen and also speak God's truth, *in love,* over you. Someone who will console you and let you cry on their shoulder and also tell you that God is good, that God is holding you, and that God is working everything out for your good!

Chapter 5

Marathon, not a sprint

My test results came back after being analyzed after surgery. My cancer was Invasive Ductal Carcinoma, and was HER2-. Which was also a good sign of possibly not needing chemo. I was beginning to feel encouraged, healing well, and in my head I thought I was done. I knew there was another final test that hadn't come back yet (completely ruling out chemo); but, I was so convinced it was going to come back "no chemo needed" because of how well everything was going. After all, I'd been able to witness something incredible during surgery, so I thought, "This was it, this is what God wanted me to see". But, "His ways are not our ways, nor His thoughts our thoughts".

The call came in and this time I was floored. I was actually at stage 3, both lumps were 1.7cm and both were cancerous (we hadn't been sure about the second tumor prior). Although they removed all of it, because it had been growing more rapidly than we thought, I would now need chemo to make sure there were no cancer cells hanging out in my blood stream waiting to attach themselves elsewhere. I felt like someone had punched me in the gut. My head was spinning and I could barely speak to finish the conversation with my doctor. Chemo! All I could think to ask was, "Am I going to lose my hair?". I'll never forget the sound in her voice when she said "Yes". It was filled with so much feeling and sounded as though she was crying with me.

It was many days of trying to remember that God still had a plan. But, I was heart broken. This seemed to affect my entire family harder than hearing the word "cancer". My children asked, "Does this mean you won't have curly hair?". Before, all they saw was mommy laying in bed and walking slowly. They would applaud me whenever I came down the stairs. But this ... this was going to be very visible, and very long.

Again I was faced with more decisions. I was offered two types of chemo. As they gave me the worst case scenarios of each treatment, none of them sounded very pleasant. BUT GOD ... there was one that stood out to me because of the words, "could cause heart issues". Well, a few months back, my Papa had died of heart issues, and again, I believe this was God's way of steering me toward the treatment I needed.

It was so much harder to shake the terrified feelings than I'd ever experienced. It was during this time that I remembered that even Jesus asked in the garden, "Let this cup pass from me. Nevertheless not my will, but thine be done". I could feel this so deeply in my soul! Then, my pastor and his wife came to visit and pray with us before my first treatment. He told me that Jesus had already gone to the door of the infusion center and back. I remembered also that God always gives us the strength right when we need it. A couple days before treatment, I was laying in bed trying to breathe, keep focused on Jesus and remember truth. Then I realized that God was already flowing through my veins. I had asked Jesus into my heart when I was 8 years old, and remembering the truth that His Spirit takes up residence inside of me, I realized that this was no surprise to my Savior and He already knew the outcome.

The day of treatment came and I was ready: physically, emotionally and spiritually. It's a very long process just to get the infusion started. They get the needle in, draw blood and send you back out to wait. Then, they call you back to get your vitals, and again you wait. They wait for your blood work to come back to make sure your body can handle the chemo. Finally, they call me back for the infusion. For some reason, they had it in their notes that I was pregnant (which I knew was not the case), so they had me do a pregnancy test just to be on the safe side. I'm thankful for how careful they are, but sheesh, it's a process. Sure enough everything came back ... not pregnant. Now we can finally get started! As the infusion starts to go in, the nurse waits to see if I have any reaction. Well, sure enough, in less than a minute I start to feel pressure in my chest. The nurse stops the infusion immediately, but not before I black out. I feel a ton more pressure in my chest that moves to my throat, and I feel as though I am being strangled and my face is swelling up. All I hear in the background is a bunch of rushing around, nurses calling my oncologist and I hear the word "EpiPen". I was aware this could happen from other friends who have also walked this journey. For one of my friends, they had slowed it way down and gave her a steroid shot. I thought that's what would happen for me. My oncologist told me it looked like I was allergic to the preservative in the chemo they gave me. I don't remember everything she said, but it was starting to sound an awful lot like I would be going home without treatment. I asked my oncologist, "Can't you try again?" (after they gave me more Benadryl and steroids). She said, "No, you don't understand. We have a scale we go by based on your reaction. You were on the dramatic end. We're not trying again today." Talk about frustrated and confused. I was ready. I went through hours of prep work only to go home without even getting across the start line! On top of that, instead of four treatments over twelve weeks, it'll now be twelve treatments - one every week.

Isn't this just like life sometimes? We think we have our act together ... we have the perfect mindset, and yet things still don't happen the we think they should. But again, "His ways are higher than ours". I'm convinced Tim was right when he said immediately afterward, "I believe God was blocking it". I'd known God was flowing through my veins and I had asked that His will be done after all. I believe I needed to choose this treatment to get to the treatment that was right for me. Yes it's inconvenient and frustrating. Especially as I'm sitting here writing this chapter with four treatments left (the original amount of treatments I was supposed to have).

The next day I was still feeling a bit of repercussions from the chemo. I had a tiny bit of pressure in my chest, but as the day went on, it began to increase with each steroid pill I was supposed to continue taking. By evening and after taking my last steroid pill, it got worse ... fast! Since we live an hour from the hospital and didn't want to wait too long considering my restricted breathing, we called the doctor and he told us to head to the ER right away. By the time we got there, my face had swollen again. It wasn't nearly as bad as the day of treatment, but the ER doctors rushed us right back. After more Benadryl and being monitored for a while, we got home late that night. This event was hard for my mind to process. I understood cancer, I understood surgery, and even chemo ... but why this? This felt like unnecessary pain because I couldn't see what God was doing.

Friends let me tell you ... sometimes things happen because God has a plan; other times it's just life. Things aren't going to go smoothly just because you keep your eyes fixed on Jesus. He absolutely gives you the strength to get through difficulties, but sometimes these things just happen and we may never understand why. This is hard to stomach, especially when you're deep in the throws of a trial that you don't understand; but, continuously remind yourself to trust God's heart. Philippians 1:6 "He (God) who began a good work in you, WILL carry it on to completion." Romans 8:28 "God works EVERYTHING together for good to those who love Him."

The next day, Tim and I were reading a devotional that said, "Sometimes when we go through hard things, we take our eyes off of Him and look for ways to serve, or the blessings of what's supposed to come after the trials." This is what I'd done. I put my eyes on what God was trying to do rather than just keeping my eyes on *Him*. I also realize sometimes things just happen. We don't always need a reason for why something happened the way it did. Sometimes it's just life. We live in a fallen world where people get sick and die. Car accidents happen. Hunger happens. Cancer happens. These things are out of our control. Many might think, "but God could have stopped this". Although that's true ... we're not God. We can't see the big picture like He can. He does give us choices ... a freewill. Years ago I thought it was just my lot in life for hard things to happen. I started to fear, "What's next?" My mind had to make the shift in thinking, "What's next" to living in each moment grateful for all the good things. My husband (who I get to call my best friend); four children that bring me joy every single day with their hugs and love; that I'm still breathing; I'm more thankful now for my curly hair than I've ever been in my life; and so many more reasons! There is always something to be thankful for and enjoy. With this mindset, it's easier to overcome the, "what-if's" and just live one day at a time ... one moment at a time. We're not promised tomorrow, but we have the choice to enjoy today for all its worth, or worry it away.

A week later, I went in for my second try at my first treatment, and this time with a plan that my oncologist, Tim, and I were more confident in and some answered prayers for wisdom about my medications. It went much better this time and I was so excited that I was able to accomplish my first treatment. A word of advice for anyone about to go through chemo. Don't wait to see how your body responds to the nausea before taking your nausea medication! Just take it and stay on top of it! Because, that's what I wish I'd done. I thought this would be like morning sickness. You start to feel sick ... then you take medication and you feel better. Uh uh!! When this hits, you can't stop it!! After a bout of constant vomiting throughout the night, I ended up going back into the infusion center to get fluids. Lesson learned!! After that one instance, it hasn't been nearly as bad as I expected. Yes, I've been tired and nauseated; but overall, I was expecting it to be so much worse.

Chapter 6

Learning to Fight for Joy

The biggest battle for me throughout my breast cancer journey has been continuously fighting for joy. It's easy to keep your eyes on Jesus when you watch the big God-moments happen, but it's harder through the mundane ups and downs of chemo treatment week after week. I was straining to keep my eyes on Jesus but becoming more and more tired of fighting. I was tired of getting a needle stuck in me every Friday. I was tired of feeling like I was missing something God wanted me to see. But here's the truth (spoiler alert), God didn't let me miss anything!

There were times when it felt like I was in the fight of my life just to stay positive. Especially three weeks into chemo treatments when I was washing my hair and big chunks started to fall out. I decided to cut my hair to my shoulders since every time I touched my hair more hair would fall out. The next washday was a nightmare. As soon as I put the shampoo in, my hair completely seized up. I worked and worked to get the knots untangled, and when I finally did, two handfuls of hair came out into my hands. And by handfuls, I mean it felt like my entire head of hair was in my hands. Just at that time, the song *Hold Me Jesus* came on my playlist. I called for Tim and asked him to cut it all off. That was one of the hardest moments of my life; I couldn't look at myself in the mirror for weeks.

It was at the halfway point I just wanted to be done ... I was tired and border line feeling sorry for myself. As if it wasn't enough to go through cancer, a mastectomy, and chemo, it felt like it was one thing after another ... I ended up battling another ear infection; a really bad back/neck crick where I couldn't even support my head; horrible bleeding because ... well ... it's that time of the month, but it lasted 2 weeks; and then, of all the nerve, I cut my finger! And yes, after all that, it was cutting my finger that broke me. But, it's a battle ... it's a choice. Do I sit in my pity party and wallow in it? No! I lift my head up and keep taking every thought captive. I keep fighting and straining my eyes to find things to be thankful for.

I started to feel myself sinking lower and lower. It felt like I was in slow-mo watching it happen, but I couldn't run away fast enough. Then, during my seventh treatment, there was a woman I overheard had cancer 18 years prior and was now going through it again. That day was her last day of chemo; she was so spunky and seemed to have such a great attitude. I thought, "if she can go through this twice and still have a good attitude, then I can stay strong through my last five treatments". It was the encouragement I needed to see. God knows when we need something tangible to set our eyes on to encourage us. We're human. I wish I could say that I can keep my eyes on Jesus without wavering, but that wouldn't be true. Very honestly, when people would comment on my smile in every picture Tim or I would post, I felt embarrassed because I knew how hard it was to smile some days. But, Jesus knows we're weak. That's why we need Him so deeply! Jesus truly has been my sustainer. That's why I've been able to continue smiling ... even when it's hard. Like right after a treatment ... my face would feel so weird and tight. I could feel the chemo rising into my head and I could feel it sitting in my throat like I drank way too much water, way too fast ... but worse; and then, it would sit there for the rest of the day. My head would spin, and I couldn't make any fast movements without getting super dizzy. Oh ... and the yucky metal taste in my mouth. Blek!

One day, in the middle of chemo, I was having a particularly hard day. It was getting harder to publicly share my journey because I'm naturally a very private person. But I felt that I needed to open my mouth and share the good, bad and ugly of my story. The reason I wanted to share ALL of it was so that God would get the glory for ALL of it. During my quiet time that day, I had escaped to my room, taken off my cap because my head needed a break, and without knowing everything that was going on in my heart, my mom came into my room with a sticky note that said, "Be Fearlessly Authentic" (that saying just so happened to come from a Dove chocolate, LOL) and stuck it on my mirror! Up until that time, my mom hadn't seen me without my cap because I was still too uncomfortable to walk around without it. She gave me the biggest hug and told me how beautiful I was. Even though I still didn't feel beautiful without my hair, I understood what she meant ... it was about more than just my hair. She encouraged me to continue sharing what God was doing and thought I needed this daily reminder. She was right! I still look at this reminder every day; it's a constant reminder to me to "Be Fearlessly Authentic" so that God gets the glory.

So far everything God has called me to do, I have the pleasure of using the delete button. When I write out posts for social media, a blog post, or a book, I can backspace as much as I want and even have my husband edit it. Or I have the blessing of the cut button while editing our podcast episodes when I've paused too long trying to figure out what I'm going to say next.

Realizing that God loves me for me, without the delete button or cutting out stutters or long pauses ... that He fearfully and wonderfully made me exactly the way He wanted, is hard to believe. I am my own worst critic. I criticize myself all the time. I still remember times when I said something that was so stupid, and I've convinced myself that the other person will never forget how stupid I was. Maybe they have forgotten, maybe they haven't ... the fact is that I'm human. I'm going to make mistakes. But, God loves me anyway. He remembers I am dust. I used to be offended by that verse. I used to think that by God remembering I am dust, He was saying, I'm *just* dust. I knew that of course I am dust and God in Heaven is holy and perfect, but recently I read that verse and it meant something different to me. God in His holiness, remembers that I am dust so therefore He doesn't expect me to be perfect. He loves me for my flaws, stutters, and awkwardness. He loves me even when I mess up. He died for my mistakes!

The beauty of my surgery story is that for once in my life I didn't care how imperfect I was. I was only doing what I heard God tell me, in my heart, to do. I spoke His name over and over, louder and louder! This is how I want to live my life everyday ...

fearlessly, authentically doing what God asks me to do. Authentically? Yes. I daily struggle with fear. It's in my DNA to have fear. So, I want to walk forward doing what God asks me to do in the middle of fear ... doing it anyway. And by walking in boldness, oddly enough, you start finding joy!

During the mundane of treatment after treatment, it was imperative for my mindset to enjoy every little thing. Taking a walk outside, drinking iced coffee, watching my children jump on the trampoline, being able to get back into yoga, watching Hallmark Christmas movies ... whatever it took. It also helped to plan a few fun things without feeling pressured in case it was a hard day to get out of bed. We did things like visiting an Apple Orchard, driving to town for ice cream, going on a date with Tim and writing this book. Keeping up with friends who cared about my cancer journey yet would also talk about daily life stuff instead of just talking about cancer all the time was also important; or, watching Dry Bar Comedy to remember to laugh. Dream a little about things in the future. Reach out to someone who is also going through a similar journey. All of these things tremendously helped keep my sanity in tact.

Chapter 7

Continuing the Fight for Joy

A few weeks after my chemo treatments ended, post trauma started to set in. Fears of the hormone treatment, "what would it do to my mind", "how would I behave", and "would I have an allergic reaction" were all flooding my mind. When I took my first pill, I began to walk on eggshells wondering every time I felt overwhelmed if I was going to turn into some sort of mad-woman. I would overthink every feeling ... EVERY everything.

I came up with the title for this book when I was in the middle of my cancer journey, but I had no idea how much I would actually have to fight for joy at the end of my cancer journey ... when everything was "supposedly" done. The post trauma and hormone treatment kicked in and it was unlike anything I'd ever felt.

I would have thoughts of, "My journey is now over, then why do I feel so lost?" or, "I don't deserve to be here anymore". I felt like my identity had been completely shaken. The hormone treatment was beginning to make me feel like I was returning to the "old Jen" after years of a battle plan for walking in grace and love. Suddenly my filter had been taken off; and although I wouldn't say anything mean or bad, things would still fly out of my mouth faster than they used to.

I felt numb! I could see and hear words of truth; but, I still felt numb. I didn't feel that fire in my belly making me want to shout God's goodness from the rooftop. I didn't even have two words to put together for a blog or podcast episode. So now what?

I thought, "My journey is over", and "I should be happy and my energy should start to return". But, I'm finding this part of my journey is harder than the cancer itself. It felt like I was always going to feel this way and I feared I'd become ineffective for Christ. I wondered if I was capable of encouraging anyone again.

You know you're in a tough spot when you'd rather go through chemo treatments than live in this entrapment of your mind! It's easy to pinpoint what's wrong with you when you have poison running through your body; you know every issue you're having is because of that. The mind doesn't work the same. I usually end up thinking, "What in the world is wrong with me?"; and, I'm tired of blaming EVERYTHING on the hormone treatment.

Here's the ugly truth about hormone treatment. If you're also being advised to take a hormone treatment, I know it's scary. I wanted to share my experiences to help you know that you are not alone and maybe give a little heads up if you're about to take it. The realization of being on this for 10 years is staggering when I realize my oldest daughter will be 20 and my youngest will be 15 when I finish. The fear of "Is this all my children will remember me as?". My experience in the last six months of taking Tamoxifen has been, insomnia, itchy legs, itchy ... down there (I told you I would get personal), getting tired really quickly and having to plan my day carefully. If I make a cake and do laundry, I need to plan for a quick and easy dinner like Grilled Cheese. I get overwhelmed very quickly at the littlest things. For example, I'll have been taking care of the kids, doing laundry, talking to a friend, and even having some quiet time in the afternoon; then by 5pm my mind is completely fried that I can't even handle the decision of what to make for dinner. Or, I'll be cooking dinner and one of the kids will come in the kitchen and ask a simple question that completely fries my brain and I freeze unable to answer a simple question. This doesn't happen constantly, but usually once a day I struggle with a similar scenario. I felt nauseated for a little while until I realized, if I took my medication around 5pm, the worst of the effects would happen while I was sleeping. My oncologist had told me to play around with different times of taking it to see what worked best for me - of course being careful not to take it too close together. I started taking it at 10pm then wanted to see how it would work if I took it earlier, so I would skip a day and take it the next day at 3pm. Then, I kept slowly pushing it back until I decided I liked 5pm best. More recently I'm starting to struggle with my bones feeling brittle. If I whack my hand against a table, it doesn't just hurt ... it's excruciating! I get back kinks a lot easier, too. I've also really been struggling with my pelvis hurting, like a more painful cramping. Sometimes it happens just because I crossed my legs or I've been sitting on a hard chair, but mostly when I have to go to the bathroom. Also, the bleeding got way more intense during that time of the month, but usually only lasts 3-5 days. I personally haven't dealt with hot flashes yet, but I've heard that is a common side effect as well.

Again, ultimately God knows your body better than you do. I've weighed the pros and cons of hormone treatment and ultimately went with my oncologist's recommendation. Although currently I'm getting so tired of all this, I just want to throw it in the trash,

I also understand that I made my choice based on what I felt my doctor advised me to do as well as what I felt peace about.

I remind myself of this question daily ... "What is truth?". The truth is that if I'm not dead, God's not done with me. I am not my feelings. Sit in Jesus' presence and take the weight off that I need to "hurry up and heal"; and instead, fall straight into the arms of Jesus. Put all the weight on Him. He can handle my pain. He doesn't get impatient with me because He remembers I'm dust and that I need Him. God wouldn't have given me a voice only to take it away again. He's stretching my muscles. He sees me struggle, but He won't allow it to crush me. This is part of my journey; it's still part of my story. God didn't say "The End" after chemo and then walk away. He's still right here. I continue to remember truth. I speak it over and over again in my mind. I continue to turn on my worship music and surround myself with friends that will also speak truth over me.

In Psalm 56:8 NLT it says, "You keep track of all my sorrows. You have collected all my tears in your bottle. You have recorded each one in your book."

This verse has been a huge comfort to me realizing no matter how many times I cry (and trust me, my bottle must be HUGE) God knows. He sees. He cares. Even when I don't feel like He sees ... He's right there!

I read the other day that we will often pray for God to be close to us (I'm guilty of this). But, we need to realize that God IS ALWAYS with us. If you have asked Jesus into your heart, then He's dwelling inside you. Instead, we need to pray, "Lord, open my eyes that I may see that you are near". I believe we just need to change our perspective. Instead of believing that God walked away, realize it's our own mindset that needs to change. The realization that He is *always* near. Nothing escapes Him! Not even your silent tears.

Chapter 8

Healing

Healing takes time. Just as your body needs time to heal after surgery, your mind needs time to heal, too. I'm guilty of trying to hurry up the process. If I could just read the right verses, sing the right songs at the right time, read the right books, or pray the right prayer with the right heart attitude everything would be better. But, God is not standing off in the distance tapping His watch wishing you would hurry up so you can be effective. God is patient, loving and kind. Just like our bodies take time to heal, so do our minds and hearts. We can't rush the process, and we're not going to heal sooner by doing "just the right steps". Rest. Abide. Allow yourself the time and headspace to heal. It can be frustrating when you're afraid your family will get frustrated with you and get tired of waiting for you to heal. But, hold them close, and just as they are giving you the grace to walk through this, give yourself grace, too. Healing can look very different for each person. Remind yourself that you have as long as it takes.

I've tried to fight the feelings of being overwhelmed in my own strength, and by the end of the day, I'm completely exhausted and tired of fighting. No, you don't want to just give up and say, "I don't care what I say, or what I do; this is just the way things are now". Rather, picture yourself falling into Jesus' arms and letting *Him* have full control. Fight with verses and take thoughts captive, but let God do the exhausting work. Take time away if you start to feel anger or frustration rising up. Pause and take a deep breath before you say something you wish you hadn't. Take it to God, and ask God to fill your mouth with His words.

One day, I pulled out my Study Bible and was drawn to a devotional titled "Trusting God in the Midst of Misery". It talks about how Job took his eyes off the holiness of God and how we can be tempted to believe that God doesn't know our circumstances. I began to read chapters 38-41 when God is asking Job, "Where were you when I laid the foundation of the earth?". As I was reading, I realized I had forgotten just how holy God Almighty is. Instead of trying to understand why I have to live with this, I'm accepting the fact that God in Heaven knows exactly what He's doing. I'm going to take my eyes off the why and just continue focusing (as I've been saying all along) on my Creator, knowing that "His ways are higher than mine".

If you're also struggling with depression like I was, I know how scary and lonely it can be. It's like a black hole that makes you feel like everything is spinning out of control and you can't figure out how to make it stop. Things that usually make you laugh barely bring a smile to your face. You feel like your smile is fake; you almost have to force it. And I'm a smiley girl. I'll smile at a stranger who passes in the grocery store, not for any reason other than the fact that they're a human being. Now, I feel as though I'd rather be under the floor.

Something I had to remind myself of during the toughest days of depression was this - I was not wrong for having depression. It wasn't because I had done something wrong, or couldn't get my act together; it was part of my journey, too. And just as Jesus had walked with me during surgery and chemo, He was walking with me in the middle of this as well. I also understand this is something no one else can understand unless they've been through it themselves. Give others grace when they're trying to understand, and even when they try to "fix" you. They're not wrong for wanting to run to your rescue. Something that helped me understand others better was putting myself in their shoes. As much as I wouldn't wish this on them, they were wishing I didn't have to go through it.

The song, *God Wants to Hear You Sing,* has meant a lot to me. Since it's not my nature to find the good in things, this song reminds me to keep my eyes focused on Jesus, and it always brings to mind Paul and Silas singing in prison. On the other hand, if you're prone to always find the good in things and you don't typically allow yourself to feel sadness or grief, this song might not mean the same to you. In which case, I want to remind you that it's ok to sit quietly with Jesus when you don't want to sing. There is a time and place for everything.

I remember one day when I woke up with my chest feeling tight, I knew it was going to be another battle. Instead of fighting it, I took the day to organize, watch *Hometown,* and just have some quiet time. Each day will look different. It's not necessarily what you do that matters; but rather, doing something different every once in a while. Take a day to go shopping, go on a hike, or stick your toes in the sand. Think differently. It always helps, even if it's just to get one day of reprieve.

Right now, I'm continuing to experience feelings of depression. Even after what God did to heal me (more on that story later). It's easy for me to go back to thoughts of "just muscle my way through to keep my eyes on Jesus", "read the right verses", or "sing the right songs at just the right time and I'll get better again". However, when I live in the fact that the point isn't to "hurry up and get better", but rather just being ok with sitting in Jesus' presence. Knowing God can still use me, He still loves me, and He's not walked away from me takes the pressure off! It allows me to actually *enjoy* His presence; not force myself into His presence. As I've mentioned before, it's falling back into His loving and caring arms. God is still good in the middle of cancer! God is still good in the midst of depression! God is still good even if you're about to walk through the "valley of the shadow of death" because who's waiting on the other side for you? Jesus himself, saying, "Well done, my good and faithful servant"!

No matter what you're facing or how hard your journey may be, one thing I want *abundantly* clear is that JESUS LOVES YOU ... ALL of you!! You are safe in His arms! When you get the dreaded call that you have cancer ... He is there. When you wake up at 3 am to get prepped for surgery ... He is there. When the IV gets started for your first chemo treatment ... He is there. When your hair begins to fall out ... He is there. When you are getting dressed into one of those "beautiful" robes to start your first radiation treatment ... He is there. When you are three treatments in and you're just plain tired ... He is there. When you've been pronounced cancer free and then the reality of everything you've just gone through starts to overwhelm you ... He is there. If you get the news that your cancer is terminal ... He is there. He is there in the mundane moments and in the hard and heavy moments. Why? Because God IS love! It's not just an attribute of God, it's who He is!

Part 2

Lessons In
The Journey

Chapter 9

The Truth About Fear

In the middle of breast cancer, I asked a question on social media: "What would you all like to know most about my cancer journey?". The greatest number of responses were how to deal with the fear. As I've mentioned previously, we need to realize that feeling fear is not wrong ... it's what happens in your next thought that counts. Are you going to give in to fear, or are you going to choose to look up and let God guide you through? I absolutely felt fear throughout this journey. The second I felt fear creep in, my battle plan was singing a song, saying my favorite verse (Isa. 43:1-2), and speaking Jesus' name. It didn't matter how many times I had to do this. The point is to keep doing it over and over ... as many times as it takes. Every other minute if you have to. And, if it feels like it's about to overwhelm you, cry out to God and ask, "What do I do?". For me, there was one night this happened. All that day I did my battle plan (focused on my verses, sang songs, took a walk ... whatever I needed in that moment); but, by evening, it was beginning to overtake me. I cried out to God and said, "I'm trying, please help me!". Immediately, I remembered my journal I'd occasionally written in since the beginning of this journey. I started reading where I'd just had my biopsy and was scared about surgery. I was scared about what my body would look like and how I would feel as a wife. I'd been shaking from removing my last Band-aid after the biopsy ... but now, I was scared about starting chemo. I was afraid it would mess up my mind so much that I would always feel like a "crazy" woman, or that my hair wouldn't grow back. I didn't know what the "new" Jennifer would be like. I'd worked so hard at being a happy mommy, choosing gratitude and looking for the positive in things - completely changing the way I took care of my kids and how I talked to Tim. As I sat there thinking about those fears I had after my biopsy, I recalled everything God had done for me! I was now eight weeks post-surgery and remembered the ways He had been there and showed me His glory in that situation! I could look at my body NOW and only feel gratefulness! The song *Scars* has taken on a whole new meaning for me. I realized if God showed up for me at the time of my surgery, He would be there again ... ready to use me in a whole new way "exceeding, abundantly, above and beyond all I could ask or think". Do you see what God did there? He led me to my journal to glance back at what He'd already done! Not only did the fear vanish; but, I was also more courageous and bold than I felt before. A renewed vigor came over me to keep getting back up and to keep on fighting!

Fear was very real, especially in the last few treatments. I was expecting something to go wrong. I had fear every week that my numbers wouldn't come back good enough to get that week's treatment. But, even after the God moment of my church coming and praying over me before my final treatment (more on that story later), the fear was REAL! It made it tougher because this was the week before Thanksgiving, and if I wasn't able to get this treatment, I would have to wait until the week after Thanksgiving. Although these fears were valid, I had to take each thought captive and make them obedient to Christ. Not think too far ahead. Just one day ... one treatment at a time.

Praise Jesus, my numbers still looked good and I was able to proceed with my LAST CHEMO TREATMENT!! I got to ring the bell that day and boy did I wish I could hug those nurses! God really blessed me halfway through my treatments with switching from a large cancer facility that did all infusions to a smaller more intimate facility that was strictly for breast care. It was much more like a family. I always had the same nurses and got to know them and love them. I messaged my family that I was DONE! They all rejoiced with me over text; but, my sisters surprised me by traveling in to celebrate! All the kids made signs to line the driveway that read "No Mo Chemo!" and they made an adorable cake! It was the most priceless gift for me to get to spend that moment with my family! Of course the final treatment hit me hard, but I was still able to enjoy Thanksgiving and was blessed to make our special meal.

There will be days when you're feeling fearful or overwhelmed and all you need is rest. Or, maybe you need to get out of the house and walk through a hiking trail, go shopping ... whatever it is that will help you feel refreshed. Something that worked yesterday, might not work today. So, always make sure that the second you feel your body tense, chest tighten, and head spin ... take a deep breath and ask yourself, "What do I need right now?" Maybe you haven't spent time with God; maybe you need fresh air; maybe you need to play with your kids; or maybe you need to get in the kitchen and bake cookies. Jesus knows your body better than you do. Don't forget that Jesus has never left you and never will. Tell Him what you're feeling. He doesn't get tired of you ... quite the opposite actually. He IS your very best friend. He IS your strength! He IS your rock! He IS your healer! He IS your helper! He IS a ring of fire around you! Have you heard that song, by the way? If not, go find "The God Who Sees" on YouTube. You're welcome!

Chapter 10

Support System

Throughout this journey, I learned the power of community! I've lost count of all the people who brought meals, cards, flowers, gifts, and even gas cards. So many people would ask what they could do to help. All the feelings of gratitude were overwhelming. Honestly, with the outpouring of messages, I didn't always know how to answer people. I love to give, but I don't always know how to receive graciously. But, because of how others were there for me throughout this process, I learned so much about how to be a friend to others, how to serve others, and how to be more empathetic towards others.

Along with the huge amount of support came the messages from well-meaning people giving advice. For this girl who is a people-pleaser, it was especially hard for me to take the advice with a grain of salt. So many people are also walking this journey. It seemed like just about everyone knew someone they wanted me to talk to. I want to encourage you not to feel like you have to talk to EVERYONE who's gone through cancer. I had to remember that God would put the ones in my path I needed to walk this journey with. For example, I would get a message saying, "God told me I'm supposed to get in this boat with you" and then they'd message me religiously asking how I was really doing and actually *really* be there (not just say they were and never check in). I have the tendency to message back giving the best case scenario - the good stuff - and shy away from sharing the bad news. I don't like talking to people when I'm down because I've had the feeling that I need to back away from others when I'm discouraged and then come back when I feel better. But, praise Jesus for the friends that still wanted to call and message when they could tell I was down. Another example was one friend jumped on FaceTime the second I cut my hair off while I was in the middle of ugly crying because she wanted to be there in that moment, through those feelings with me.

So, how do you deal with all the advice and well-meaning comments from family, friends, acquaintances and even strangers? There will be many well-meaning people on this journey, but sometimes it's necessary to take some parts of the advice and let go of other parts. Tuning out the comments on social media at times or taking a break from constant text messages is also healthy. I remember one person saying, "You have such a tremendous mission field to every nurse you meet". In reality, it was hard to carry on a conversation with my nurses because they were so busy. I put so much unnecessary pressure on myself that it took my eyes off what God wanted MY story to look like. And although, yes, I could still be a light to every nurse, doctor, and patient I saw, it didn't mean that's the mission field God intended for me. Your journey will look completely different from mine and that's the beautiful thing. God has a special, unique, custom-made journey just for you and He is going to walk you through every step of the way. Yes, you can have a mission field right in the middle of this journey, but something I had to continually remind myself was to look at Jesus, not the mission field.

The support of your family is so key. There were some very precious moments throughout my recovery from surgery. The attentiveness of my sweet husband, and the fact that my oldest daughter (Nicole) wanted to help in the cleaning of my drains made me feel so loved. I was so proud of how she handled it ... not squeamish at all like her mother. LOL! Tim, my mom, and the kids brought me coffee in bed. The card games along with the many gentle hugs and kisses from my sweet kiddos sure did this Mama's heart good. My mom would cook supper and we'd eat up in our bedroom each night. We'd have movie nights and watch shows like *Andy Griffith* until I was strong enough to go downstairs.

Nicole had already talked about being a nurse when she got older and was studying a book on the human body that her Aunt Rachel (who is a nurse) had given her. She shared one night that she felt called to be a nurse because of my cancer diagnosis. And can I just pause a moment and give a huge shout out to all the amazing nurses!! They truly are angels on earth and I have loved every one that I have come in contact with ... well, most of them if I'm being completely honest (some did NOT know how to find my veins). But, I appreciate all of them just the same!

I had to choose to rest. Although my family wouldn't let me do a lot of work around the house, sometimes I would beg them to let me make dinner or do the laundry because I needed to feel useful, LOL! So, it wasn't always physical rest that I needed, but often mental rest! I didn't need to constantly be a spiritual pillar; sometimes I just needed to BE. I had to realize it was ok to shut my phone off and completely rest. And at other times, get in the kitchen (my happy place) and make a cake or cookies.

The Sunday before my final treatment I woke up completely exhausted. It takes a lot of internal energy for this introvert to record podcast episodes, write blog posts and all the other things that I feel called by God to do. So, when I woke up that morning, I decided to stay in introvert mode for a little bit and read. I picked up *Strong, Brave, Loved* by Holley Gerth and was encouraged by the verse, "we are surrounded by so great a cloud of witnesses ..." It got me thinking about my brother David and Papa up in Heaven ... honestly a little jealous of them getting to be with Jesus! I opened my window and began to pray over my friends when I saw one of the deacons from our church walking below my window followed by another from our small group. Soon after, I heard our entire small group surround our home and begin to pray over me and my family! WOW! What an encouragement this was to me and my family. It gave me the final push I needed to cross the finish line!

Besides friends who said, "I believe I'm supposed to get in this boat with you", and our church coming to pray around our home, there were so many individuals God placed in our lives who had already been through cancer and they knew what to tell me at just the right time. We were in awe of how God had moved us to this place for such a time. God also placed amazing people in Tim's work that were there for him and were adamant he take time off whenever it was needed. He was able to drive me to every appointment and infusion. I remember Tim had written the verse, Exodus 14:14, over his desk,

"The Lord will fight for you, you need only be still." The day I found out I was supposed to get my rushed biopsy the very next day, Tim called his Senior Vice President letting him know because he had a bunch of internal Zoom meetings and such scheduled for that day. A few minutes later, Tim's phone blew up with notifications, "meeting cancelled, meeting cancelled, meeting cancelled". Not only were they supportive, but they were fighting for us!

There will be times where you will need discernment in your support system. Not everyone who walked this journey needs to be *in* this journey with you. Listen to the Spirit. You don't have to take all the advice. Don't force a fit. Be open, but discerning. Live in grace and gratitude!

Chapter 11

A note to those walking alongside someone with cancer

Although I've not had any immediate family go through cancer, I've experienced my family and friends walk alongside me, graciously pray over me, talk with me and take amazing care of me. I believe it's just as hard for you to watch your loved one walk through cancer as it is to go through it yourself, because you can't do anything to take it away. So, I would like to encourage you to find someone you trust and can talk to; and, don't forget to take care of yourself. Take some time to walk away for a little while and do something you enjoy. As someone who has watched my loved ones suffer on my behalf, I've witnessed how imperative it is to keep yourself whole and healthy: emotionally, spiritually, and physically. Along with my own observations, I asked each of those closest to me what helped and encouraged them and have included that in this chapter.

What I needed most from my loved ones were hugs (lots and lots of them) and a listening ear. So many other things were a HUGE blessing. Like my mom taking over the household chores, dinner, and watching the kids while Tim and I went for appointments and infusions. And then many other things were done for me - things I would've never thought about but were a huge blessing! Friends flying across country to visit me, and my sisters and friends sending me care packages just to make me smile. The phone calls where we didn't just talk about cancer but also about regular life stuff and things that made me laugh (although they'd allow me to vent and say how much cancer sucks). It meant a lot to me when my family would cry on my shoulder and be mad about my cancer. When they would lean on me for support, it gave me purpose as well and showed how much they cared about me. I have to say, I could have lived without that face app where you can change your physical appearance. My sweet husband was trying to be supportive and wanted to shave his head for me. So he thought if I could see what he'd look like without hair before he shaved it, I would be fine with it. That didn't go over very well, LOL! But, he was trying and that's what meant a lot to me. A good question in general might be to ask, "What would serve you best right now?"

After asking my close family and friends what encouraged *them* throughout this journey, these were their responses. My children said it was praying a lot, talking about everything going on, or seeing me talk to my friends because they could tell it cheered me up. Also, helping me, choosing thankfulness, picking flowers, doing other special things for me, and reading verses that were applicable to this situation. Tim said it was talking to someone else who's walked this journey and staying engaged even though your world feels like it's spinning. When you decide not to isolate yourself and continue to show up, you end up forming more friendships and becoming more encouraged. He emphasized you DON'T have to be strong; it's ok to be weak. It encouraged him to watch the kids make cards and pray for me. He says, "It's definitely about staying connected and doing it together as a family." My mom said what encouraged her was being able to help and stay involved. Music was also a huge encouragement for her and the many many hugs. My sisters said that it was realizing God loves me more than anyone else possibly could, and He would only allow what's best ... even if it's hard and doesn't make any sense from a human perspective. And knowing HE is in complete control brought them peace! Also, having music playing throughout the day especially when I was heavy on their hearts was a huge encouragement - a favorite was "Fear Not Tomorrow, God is Already There" by the Collingsworth family. They say, "Turn worried thoughts into prayers, and then don't wait to be asked to do something ... jump in and find some way to help." Putting feet to their worries and finding ways to act was very healing and encouraging to their hearts as well as mine. My friends said it was every morning waking up and putting it in God's hands. One said it was allowing herself to have total faith in the fact that God is good, no matter the outcome. Also focusing on doing everything she could to be helpful and bring joy during that season. That took the focus off of fear and put her desire to do something to good use.

As the one walking through cancer, I want you to know that you are an important part of this journey! Don't be afraid to let your feelings show! You are extremely loved and just as important in God's eyes! He sees you too! As I said earlier, I believe it's just as hard to watch your loved one walk through this as it is to walk through it yourself. You are seen! You are important! You are loved! And I want to thank you from the bottom of my heart for the love, prayers, and actions you give so willingly!

Chapter 12

Tips and Tricks I've Learned

I had a friend, Amy, that was my angel on earth. She sat down with me over coffee, told me her story of breast cancer without leaving out the hard stuff. She didn't sugar coat anything which I was grateful for. But, she also told me I was going to get through this with the help of Jesus. She gave me ideas that would help me after surgery and alerted me about things to expect from chemo. I'm going to pass this information along to you with some helpful ideas from others, as well as some things I've learned to hopefully help you feel more prepared and set your mind at rest.

Since I was having a mastectomy with tissue reconstruction, I could hardly use any upper body muscles after surgery. You have to be careful how you stand up, lay down, twist and turn, etc. So, the things I found to be most helpful in preparation were:

- Elevated toilet seat (if you're having tissue reconstruction)

- Chair for the shower

- Hand-held shower head with hose/mount

- Loose fitting, soft pants

- Blousy shirts (something with pockets is best so you have a place to put your drains. The trickiest thing, by far, was figuring out what to wear with the drains)

- Flowy dresses (after the drains have been removed)

- Soft bra's with no wire

- Rolled gauze (to lay across your incision, if you're having tissue reconstruction)

- Books (Both fiction and non-fiction. Some non-fiction that were encouraging were "Unexpected" by Christine Caine, "The Power of Jesus' Names" by Tony Evans, "Peace" by Becky Thompson, and "Strong, Brave, Loved" by Holley Gerth), crossword puzzles, and movies to keep you occupied in the long weeks of recovery.

The things I found most helpful during chemo were:

- Water jug (because you need to drink LOTS of water)

- Bag filled with: blanket, crosswords, snacks, and books for treatment days

- *Liquid IV* (Hydration multiplier and electrolyte booster)

- *Juice Plus* (Daily vitamins that my oncologist gave me permission to continue taking because it's strictly fruits and vegetables, but make sure you check with your oncologist.)

- *As I Am* Co-wash (My hair became extremely dry and fragile about a week into treatments, so you definitely don't want anything too harsh. I also never completely lost all of my hair, although it was incredibly sparse, so I continued to use it all the way through treatments.)

- Caps or a wig (Try to make it as fun as you can. I loved the caps that were braided across the top that I purchased from Amazon)

I also encourage you to get a good skin care routine, if you don't already. When I lost my hair, it was important for me to have nice skin. Paint your nails, if you want. Start a project that gets you outside of yourself and do something for someone else. Do puzzles or paint by number. Make a gift basket for someone else going through cancer. Keep a journal of all your feelings and what God is doing through you. (As I've previously mentioned, this is great to be able to look back and see what God has done). Do small things that give you something to look forward to.

After chemo, a whole new set of things have been life savers for me because of growing my hair back, healing mentally and starting Hormone Treatment:

- *Kerotin* vitamins (Make sure to check with your doctor before you take ANY supplements. What works alongside my medication may not be ok with yours.)

- Headbands (These made me feel a bit more girly after I was ready to take the caps off.)

- Melatonin (Because my hormone treatment was causing insomnia, but again check with your oncologist first.)

- *Curlsmith* Scalp Stimulating Booster

- *Skin Balm Apothecary* hair oil

- Keeping Kleenex's in every room of the house, LOL! (I mean, I've always been a cryer, but this is something else entirely, haha!)

- A new worship playlist (what was encouraging during the thick of surgery and chemo kept putting me back in that mindset while I was trying to heal mentally and found that changing my music from encouraging music to simply worship was what I needed.)

- The book *Don't Give The Enemy A Seat At Your Table* by Louie Giglio was great to read while I was in the midst of depression

Remember to laugh and just enjoy life. I have the tendency to be very serious minded. I'm always thinking would God be pleased with that thought, music, movie, etc. I have to remind myself even though I want to always bring God glory, I also need to lighten up and just have fun. You only get to live once and if you're in the middle of cancer then it has definitely crossed your mind that life is short. Enjoy every moment to the fullest.

Chapter 13

Look Up

I've mentioned "Look up" and "Keep your eyes on Jesus" throughout this book; now, I want to really dive deep into these statements because together they're the overarching message of my entire journey. This is what I believe God really wanted me to see and what I believe He wants me to "speak up" about for the rest of my life.

As I've mentioned previously, once I started the hormone treatment, beside dealing with the side effects, depression was definitely the hardest part. It's one thing to listen to someone who is going through depression (you try to listen, understand and be there for them), but it's something entirely different to walk through it yourself. Learning to deal with a chemical inside my body has been a struggle. I had begun to think my battle plan that's always worked for every situation doesn't apply to me because I have a chemical that's taking over my mind. But one day,

I'd had enough of depression! I didn't want to live in this darkness any longer! I looked out the window, up at the sky, and said, "NO!" ... "Jesus, get me out of this. I know I'm not the only person who suffers from this. Give me the recipe to get out, so I can help other women get out of this as well!"

I immediately felt I needed to research what "Abide" meant. It was my word for the year that I'd chosen in January of 2021. I had a general idea of what the word meant, but I had never actually researched it. What I found has changed me! An article by *Desiring God*, describes it this way: "To abide is believing, trusting, savoring, resting and receiving". The words savoring and receiving really jumped out at me. I hadn't ever considered those words as describing abide. Consider the scripture that says, "I am the vine, you are the branch". Whatever comes through the vine goes directly to the branch. If we're hungry, He feeds us (daily bread), if we're thirsty, He gives us water (living water). Whatever our need, He provides and satisfies. I'm not saying we'll never have fear again or look at the waves around us; but now, instead of feeling like there's no hope, we can KNOW that NO MATTER the circumstances, we simply must keep our eyes on Jesus! He can overcome ANYTHING!!

Abide! Fully trust, fully rest, fully savor, fully believe, actively receive and be in constant fellowship with

Jesus. This is easier said than done, but my heart is crying out for you to understand the freedom that you CAN live in!

Abide means to fully trust. Trust that even when you don't see how a life circumstance could possibly turn out good, "God works everything out for good to those who love Him." It might not turn out exactly the way *you* wanted it to, but it *will* turn out for the good of God's glory.

Abide means to fully rest. This means laying down EVERY care, EVERY fear, EVERY bit of anxiety. Lay down all the weight of everything that keeps you awake at night and picture yourself resting at Jesus' feet.

Abide means to savor. Think about a piece of cake that was absolutely divine and you wanted to savor every bite. Or maybe a moment spent with a child or best friend and you wanted to savor every second spent with them because it was such a sweet time. Do you savor Jesus? Every ounce of love and grace that He has poured into you; do you savor every moment you sit with Him in sweet fellowship?

Abide is the act of receiving. Receive everything Jesus has to offer. Remember the analogy of the vine and the branch? Everything that Jesus has to offer is right in your reach. It flows straight from Him to you if you are connected to His power source. All the power, love, truth, daily bread and living water that flows from Him, you have access to.

Abide means being in fellowship with Jesus. Yes, read your Bible and pray. But it's so much more than that! Have constant communication with Him. Think about your best friend that you always want to share the good, bad and ugly with. Have that relationship with Jesus, but even closer. The second you wake up, are you reaching for your phone or do you feel like you're picking up a conversation with Jesus that you left off from the night before? The second you have to make a tough decision at work, or your kids just made a bad choice and you have to decide how to handle it, is your first thought to ask God, "What do I do?"

Throughout that week of dwelling on what abide meant. God also gave me three things - my recipe:

1. Take every thought captive
2. Put your eyes on Jesus
3. Remember who God is

By living out these three things over the course of a week, I was changed! I *literally* took every thought captive and made it obedient to Christ. This means that with EVERY. SINGLE. THOUGHT. I compared it to the truth in God's word. If I had the thought, "I will never be used by God", I threw it out and replaced it with, "He who began a good work in you, will carry it on to completion". If I thought, "I don't deserve to be here anymore; maybe it would've been better if cancer had taken me", I remembered, "If I'm not dead, God's not done".

When I would feel fear, depression overtaking me, or my chest began to tighten, I would remember these truths and then I'd immediately put my eyes on Jesus. I would picture His nail-driven hands or feet. I would imagine myself laying on His chest and feeling His love pour into me.

I would remember who God is! I read through Job 38-41 with tears streaming down my face as I read, "Where were you when I laid the foundation of the earth? Tell me if you have understanding. Who determined its measurements - surely you know!" I remembered just how holy and powerful God Almighty is! I remembered, it's not about me ... it's all about JESUS!

After the healing from depression, I have had moments where fear would creep in. I would try really hard to do the recipe God gave me and wonder, "Why is it not working this time?" That's when I had to stop trying and remember, it's not about "doing" the recipe, it's about falling into His arms, casting out the lies in my mind and replacing them with truth, and instead of forcing my eyes on Jesus, just fall back *into* Jesus! That's the ultimate trust exercise, right?! Falling backward into your friend's arms and hoping they catch you. With God, there is no *hoping* that He will catch you. HE WILL catch you! Not only that, but this allows Him to come into your situation and take control.

If you're going through cancer or walking alongside someone who has cancer; or perhaps this book has found you and you are neither of these but are in just as much of a struggle (with fear, anxiety or a life circumstance that seems like it's winning and you're losing), my prayer for you is that you would find peace in the midst of this storm! I pray that you feel the tenderness of our loving Savior wrapped around your heart!

What are you choosing to look at? The waves around you? Or Jesus who has the power to calm the waves or hold you as He rides the waves with you?! 2 Chronicles 20:12 says, "We are powerless ... we don't know what to do, but our eyes are on you"! Do you have an escalated attention to who God is? Are you intentional about identifying what IS truth? Do you meditate on truths more than the situation you are facing? Yes, we see the struggle, but then we pivot and keep our eyes on Jesus!

What I desire for you to see throughout my story more than anything is JESUS! I want you to know that He is GOOD! He is LOVE! He is with you!

A Note From Jennifer

This entire journey for me can be summed up in one word. Thankfulness! Thankful to be alive. Thankful for doctors and nurses. Thankful for family and friends. Thankful to be entrusted with this breast cancer journey. And thankful most of all that God showed me once again He will never leave me nor forsake me. That He holds me ... even when I don't feel it!

Thankfulness has not always been my first response. Like when we lived without running water for 7 months. Yes, I'm thankful now for that experience; but, that wasn't my initial response. Maybe you're thinking, "How could I possibly be thankful for cancer?" But you see, God has a track record with me. I've seen Him do so many incredible things in my life ... how can I *not* trust Him and choose to be thankful?!

Even now, as I finish this book, I've found out at my yearly mammogram that my cancer has returned

... but, I trust Him! It feels so much different this time around because of everything you just read. God's track record with me through my first cancer diagnosis was this - He was there! And I know that "He will NEVER leave me or forsake me!" There's not nearly as much fear because God got me through once, He'll get me through it again! But this time around, I'm determined cancer doesn't get front seat! It's going to take the back seat to everything God is calling me to do. Yes, I will absolutely be following all my doctors suggested treatments (which this time will be lumpectomy and radiation), but I decided to register to become a certified life coach the same day the doctor called telling me I have cancer again. Why? Because I feel called to do this and I'm not going to let cancer get me down!

I don't know what I would do without having God as my strength. The only way I can continue going through this journey is because of my Lord and Savior Jesus Christ! I would like to take this moment and ask if you have a personal relationship with Jesus? Jesus paid the ultimate sacrifice because He loves *you*!! He died on the cross, took the penalty for all the wrong things we've done and placed it on Himself. Then, He rose again to show that He has the victory over death! He took away the sting of death! All we have to do is invite Him to take up residence inside of us and we get to live for eternity with HIM!

That gives me goose bumps every time! To think that the God who created the universe, keeps the planets and stars in place, made the beauty that we get to enjoy all around us ... wants to have a relationship with *me* ... it just astounds me! How could I not want Him in every part of my life?!

Let me also say that accepting Jesus is not a way to escape hard things. We will still experience hard things such as cancer. The difference is Jesus gives a peace that you just can't explain, and to experience it is the greatest gift!

If you would like to talk more about having a relationship with Jesus, please email me at hooper. jend@gmail.com and I would love to talk more with you. I want you to know that God still has a plan for you. I love how Holley Gerth wrote in her book *Strong, Brave, Loved,* "Whatever the future brings, our God is still holding the pen. He is the only one who gets to write, 'The End'". In your fight for joy, I pray that you look to the One who has already fought for you!

With all my love,
Jen